# PAIN-FREE

## How to Live a Full Life

## Despite Chronic Pain

**Michele Johnson MHS, PA-C**

**The PainFree PA**

# Contents

# Introduction

Pain-free. I bet you're intrigued by the thought of being free of pain. The knowledge and inspiration you will gain from this book lies in being able to reframe your understanding of the word "pain-free." As a fibromyalgia patient, I have coexisted with pain nearly every day for eighteen years. Pain has taught me lessons I couldn't have learned otherwise. My reframed concept of pain-free involves living a full life despite living with chronic pain.

After returning to college at age thirty-one, I graduated with my master's degree from Duke University Medical Center as a physician assistant. My training has allowed me to travel to China on a medical delegation to learn about traditional acupuncture and herbal medicine. Later, as a practicing clinician, I witnessed doctors in Cuba provide superior health care despite limited resources. My amazing, supportive husband, Toney, and my bright and funny thirteen-year-old son, Matthew, keep me motivated to live the best life possible.

However, it wasn't always this way. At twenty-three, I sat in the corner of the disability office dressed in layers, a skullcap hiding my hair. Keeping my head down, I avoided eye contact with anyone coming in. After being laid off from my customer service position at a failing telecom company, I was on food stamps to help keep my fridge stocked. Now, sitting in the disability office, I compared my appearance to that of the other applicants in wheelchairs or carrying their oxygen tanks. The examiner called me in to check my vision and watch me complete physical tasks. She had that now familiar look on her face: the "You don't look sick" look. I recognized it immediately, I have experienced it with doctors and teachers in the past. As I expected, my denial letter came a couple of weeks later.

My mother's voice chanted in my head: "You can always pick yourself up, brush yourself off, and start all over again." She'd said that every time I made a mistake growing up. This was not the end—I just needed a plan.

Through the years, I found my strengths, and I had to use them to pull myself up over and over again. My mental and physical health have grown tremendously through my work with patients and their families. In serving others with my gifts, I have seen great gains in my own health.

*Pain-Free: Living a Full Life Despite Chronic Pain* is intended to start a conversation about thriving in spite of chronic pain and invisible illness. The victories and trials highlighted in this book will inspire you to examine what you can accomplish in your *own* life despite chronic pain. No person is an accident or placeholder; there is something unique and valuable in each of us, and we all have something to contribute to the world.

Let's explore what your life can be despite any physical limitations.

Welcome.


*Disclaimer: All cases are based on actual experiences. Some physical attributes and names have been altered to protect the privacy of the subjects.*

# Chapter 1: Invisible Pain

*"When you have an invisible disease, your sickness isn't your biggest problem. What you end up battling more than anything else, every single day, is other people."*

—*Heidi Cullinan,* Carry the Ocean

Standing outside the exam room door, I removed my white coat and set it on an empty chair in the hall. Sighing heavily, I read the next patient's visit description: "Chronic pain management." Was he seeking drugs? He was only scheduled for twenty minutes, but would it take an hour?

Deep breath! *Check you bias at the door*, I chided myself. I knew what it was like to have someone judge me before they even listened. *Remember to just listen.*

After opening the exam room door, I saw a six-foot-five black male with shoulder-length dreadlocks sitting on a chair near my desktop. Kai looked as if he didn't want to have this conversation any more than I did. After so many doctor's appointments myself, I knew that look. However, there was something more, something behind the frustration in his eyes.

After introducing myself as the physician assistant who would be taking care of him. I asked, "What brings you to see me today?" My smile was intentionally warm as I attempted to be disarming and compassionate about whatever might come out of his mouth next.

Norco, narcotic pain medication, every six hours. He couldn't figure out why it wasn't working to make him pain-free. As he talked, I watched his body movements. He had to adjust his posture every few moments, as his leg muscles tensed if in the same position for too long.

He stretched his legs along the linoleum floor, then bent his knee against the skinny black legs of his chair. He looked down at the floor or up to my writing table, never in my eyes. He wanted my help but seemed unsure if he would receive any relief at all.

Leaning in, I put my hand on his shoulder. Looking into his eyes, I asked, "What happened to you? How did this start?" His eyes sank, as if he was overcome with emotion he didn't want to show. The strong, skeptical man became vulnerable. Though it was obviously hard for him to talk about his story, I watched his body relax as he started to share it.

He described how the bullets had pierced his flesh over and over again. In total, Kai had received nine gunshot wounds. Sleeping at a friend's house, he was awakened by the pop of gunshots ringing out through the house. He had no idea what the altercation was about; unfortunately bullets can't explain that.

The metal rods now surgically implanted in his legs were made of titanium. They didn't move as easily as bones and joints, so he felt continuously uncomfortable.

After all the hospital stays and pain specialist visits, he was emotionally exhausted. Having to justify how much pain he was in served to make him relive his trauma over and over in front of strangers. He knew they judged him as a thug who likely had it coming.

Despite the various medications, surgeries, and counselors, he still had pain every single day. He had lost all hope in medical science being able to help.

Few of us have been through the challenge of rebuilding our lives after having being shot multiple times. However, the struggle of trying to live a normal life despite the presence of daily pain and the judgment of other people is very relatable.

Like Kai, many people I meet feel exasperated about explaining their pain. We explain it to our families, to our medical providers, and sometimes we find ourselves explaining it to our own mirror.

And Kai, like many of my patients, was going through emotional trauma that had never been addressed. The pain of his wounds was complicated by the pain of his fear and anxiety. However, after months of office visits, counseling, and exploring community resources, he started to need less and less medication.

He adopted meditation techniques and found more time in his schedule to exercise and spend time with his young child. As we addressed the causes of his pain and practical solutions for his needs, he flourished. His new framework became a path to living a full life despite his chronic pain.

Chronic pain has many faces and takes many shapes. It's really important to educate yourself on what you are facing.

There's so much information at our fingertips; the internet has definitely created a greater access to knowledge than ever before. However, with all the misinformation on websites, it can be very confusing trying to find solutions that work.

But by knowing the facts and myths about your condition, you can understand the symptoms common to your diagnosis, as well as what symptoms are cause for alarm. This knowledge about what you are facing is empowering and very helpful when trying to communicate with medical professionals and your family.

I had to learn what I was facing myself when I first got ill. Having several friends and family members with lupus, cancers, and other chronic illnesses, I was very nervous about the prognosis for fibromyalgia when I met my first rheumatologist, Dr. Katz.

In 2001, there wasn't a lot of information about fibromyalgia despite the three million people estimated to have the condition. Doctors were still debating if it was rooted in physical causes or mental ones. They knew that small nerves along the muscles would become "overexcited" in response to stimuli that weren't normally painful. However, many doctors believed that fibromyalgia was "all in the patient's head."

Though not fatal, fibromyalgia is a daily nemesis. It robs you of sleep, the ability to make plans with others, and the security of being able to trust your own body. This illness, invisible to those who look at me, would hurt any area of my body at any time. This was my new every day. Knowing I wouldn't die from fibromyalgia made me driven to learn how to live with it. Knowledge of what I was up against empowered me to keep moving toward my goals, one step at a time.

# Chapter 2: Mourn and Move

*"Grief is like the ocean; it comes on waves ebbing and flowing. Sometimes the water is calm, and sometimes it is overwhelming. All we can do is learn to swim."*

*—Vicki Harrison*

Falling asleep between stoplights and nearly crashing my car on the way to work were what forced me to seek medical attention. Between juggling my full-time job as a customer service representative, being a leader in the teen ministry at my church, and daily rehearsals for the annual Christmas show dance routines, my plate was full. It was reasonable to think I could be extremely tired.

Mornings were the worst. It felt as if a truck had run over me, and I had to peel myself from the concrete of my bed using all the strength I had left. It was exhausting. Coffee provided some help.

I hadn't told my family how I was feeling; they were a little distant since I'd joined the church and become on fire for Jesus. I often quoted Bible scriptures and told people how their way of living would land them in Hell. If I hadn't been so busy with work, Bible talks, leadership training, teen outings, and practicing for the show, I might have actually felt the void of not talking to my family.

I was raised with cousins who loved me like a sibling, and aunts who had permission to spank me if they saw me misbehaving. We had Christmas Eve talent shows and backyard barbecues. I missed them, but my new church home was all about saving souls and living life as a Christian in the one true church.

Nobody knew about my falling asleep at the wheel, my concrete limbs in the morning, or the needle pain in my feet when I walked.

The rheumatologist, Dr. Katz, diagnosed me with a chronic pain and fatigue illness called fibromyalgia. He then proceeded to question my exercise routine. My levels of creatine kinase (CK), an enzyme released into the blood when there's muscle damage, were more than nine times what they normally should be. He was concerned I might be in rhabdomyolysis, a sometimes life-threatening breakdown in skeletal muscle caused by direct or indirect injury, and need emergency care if I didn't stop dancing.

After the doctor told me I would have pain and fatigue every day, his next sentence took away something I loved, something that had been a source of joy on the dark days. He said I couldn't dance again. The doctor encouraged me to rest my muscles and rehydrate till I felt better.

What did you lose when you found out your pain would be chronic?

For some it's the loss of an ability, while for others it's the loss of their role in the family. It's important to acknowledge the loss.

For some, it becomes a source of bitterness and anger. The sense of loss makes them push away anyone who tries to get close. For others, the tears come daily, and the sadness of not being able to live the life you had designed for yourself is crippling.

Allow yourself to feel what you feel. Let it all come through your body and even out onto paper if that's helpful for you. This is grief. You're mourning the loss of your former ideal, your former self. When my dad passed away after an eight month battle with stomach cancer, I used therapy to help navigate the waves of grief I felt. It is the same with mourning the loss of your former or ideal self. Whatever the resource, get the help that you need. Though I will share many helpful techniques and stories of my former patients, friends, and myself, remember that you'll be writing your own story. If you haven't mourned the losses you've endured, it will be difficult to move on to create a new life and a new sense of what you can accomplish.

Disregarding the doctor's orders, I decided to dance in the show. The adrenaline must have been high, and as we reached the famous marquee of the Chicago Theatre, I felt no pain that day. Performing there was a once-in-a-lifetime experience, and I couldn't stop smiling.

Our dress rehearsal beneath the auditorium revealed the wall of autographs. Michael Jackson, Prince, and many others had scribbled their names on the curved concrete wall. I couldn't scratch my name in ink between those famous names, though I tried multiple times.

Starstruck and honored to be where I was, I discovered that my wallet had been swiped. Still, the loss of my money and identification cards couldn't curb the excitement building inside of me.

Listening backstage, I felt my heart leap repeatedly into my throat while I was awaiting my cue to come on stage. My smile, showing all thirty-two of my teeth, was fixed all night. Swing dancing with Emmanuel, the star of the number, went off without a hitch. Deep breaths calmed my anxiety as behind the curtain I awaited my next dance number.

Sweat streamed down my back and forehead as I donned a black hoodie and baggy sweatpants for the hip-hop routine at the end of the night. Our formations were tight and hard hitting. We moved as one, and the audience erupted in applause after. Exiting the stage, I found my breathing heavy and labored. My friends worried and carried me out after hearing the wheezing from my lungs when I exhaled.

Despite the joy and excitement of the performance, exhaustion overtook my body. The incessant pounding of my heart made me nervous that I could pass out at any moment. This convinced me to heed the doctor's advice: I wouldn't dance again.

Learning that my body had limits forced me to think creatively about what I could do, instead of focusing on what I couldn't do. I acted in church plays and led events for our teens. I adapted my actions to things that didn't hurt as much.

Though I mourned the loss of the possibility of dancing again, I knew I couldn't let my limitations define me. Nor should you.

How can you creatively use your knowledge and abilities to create a fulfilling life, despite your physical limitations? Mourn the losses from your illness, but the key is to not stay stuck in loss. Get moving with purpose toward what is possible and serves others.

# Chapter 3: The Right Thing, Not Just Anything

*"Doing more things faster is no substitute for doing the right things."*

*—Stephen Covey*

With so many options to control pain and inflammation, it can be difficult to know who or what treatment plan to trust. Diets, medications, and stimulators all promise to make dramatic changes in your pain. The difficulty with bringing about pain relief is that every person is different, and so responds to different treatments.

Diet can often help, as was the case for my cousin, Kiera. She called me to talk about her symptoms. This wasn't uncommon. As the medical person in the family, I was used to responding to all types of embarrassing questions that came up. This was different, though. When she started to describe the spikes in her blood pressure to the 200s, and the fact that her doctors were saying she'd had a mini-stroke, the hairs on the back of my neck stood up.

At twenty-two, Kierra was brilliant and had traveled to Europe and India to aid in disaster recovery. She didn't smoke cigarettes, drink alcohol, or do drugs. There really was no reason for her to suddenly have these alarming symptoms.

As she tried to recall her discussions with the emergency room doctors, I kept thinking about how familiar her symptoms sounded. I blurted out, "That's lupus until proven otherwise."

A year after our conversation, she was finally diagnosed with lupus. Lupus is an autoimmune disease, meaning that essentially the body attacks itself because it doesn't recognize its own cells. In her case, lupus attacked her cardiovascular system, causing high blood pressure, blood clots, and extreme fatigue.

In medical training, when we were asked a question about a disease that can take many forms and look like many others, we all knew we could say lupus and be considered on the right track. Lupus can attack any organ in the body and produce a host of symptoms. Though lupus patients look healthy on the outside, there's a war going on inside them.

After her diagnosis, my relative began to read all she could about ways to help herself. She started on a vegan diet and has slowly been able to wean herself off all medication for her lupus and blood pressure.

Pain and inflammation can be fed by the foods we choose. Plant-based diets have caused remarkable improvement in diabetes, and in autoimmune and chronic pain diseases. The science shows over and over again that this diet get results. The difficulty lies in actually eating a plant-based diet.

Our culture is about convenience and moving fast. Many don't have time to plan, shop for, and cook nutritious meals. Some of us don't have the money to buy more expensive, healthy foods, so we feed our whole house for much less money with unhealthy foods.

The first part to address in our relationship with food is to define its purpose in our lives. Food has become a focal point of celebrations, a consolation in times of sadness, and a gift of congratulations. Food has become much more than nourishment—more like a family friend.

Since our intake of food affects our weight and the load on our joints, the acid balance in our stomachs, and our moods, it's wise to be more thoughtful about what we consume. There are tons of diet and nutrition books and gurus teaching their own diets, but what has been really effective for my patients is keeping a food diary.

Starting with healthy foods you know you enjoy, look for simple meals you can plan around those items. As you incorporate these foods, log how you feel. Note your energy level, your pain, and your blood pressure or blood sugar levels if necessary.

This is your life's work, as you only get one body. Do the best you possibly can with it.

Of course, not all chronic pain illnesses are a result of inflammation or weight gain. Fibromyalgia is a nerve and muscle condition, and there is no "special diet" to dramatically reduce my pain. However, I have seen those with inflammatory arthritis and lupus make dramatic improvements. Healthier eating makes us feel well, even though it doesn't cure the illness.

Admittedly, for most of my life I have felt as if exercise is a dirty word. For someone with daily pain, it doesn't make sense to torture already pained muscles and joints. Dance was my exercise for years, but since that became dangerous for me, I had to find another outlet.

Unsure of what exercises would work well without causing excruciating pain and days of recovery, I wasn't sure where to start. The memories of a prescribed physical therapy regimen I began still plague me to this day.

Twenty years ago, physical therapy wasn't as refined as what I recommend for my patients today. The regimen resembled cruel and unusual punishment. The dark room was intended to be relaxing, but the beeping machines and bulky tools made my anxiety rise.

Bending my legs and arms in directions they didn't seem meant to go, the therapist seemed satisfied only after a joint would crack and I would moan from the pain. Each maneuver was a surprise I couldn't brace myself for. But the therapist assured me that after the agony of stretching out my muscles, I would have sweet relief from a soothing massage.

The promised massage was a TENS (transcutaneous electrical nerve stimulation) unit placed on my back to help relax my aching body. Instead of relief, it felt as though multiple birds were pecking at my already inflamed muscles. Most days I went home feeling worse than when I arrived. I usually spent the day off between physical therapy days in bed as a recovery period, a hiatus until the torture was to start again.

This prescribed therapy made me feel like a failure at the simple task of moving my muscles. For years, I thought there was no exercise regimen I could handle without having excruciating pain afterward. I was so wrong.

Yoga and tai chi have been great additions to my exercise toolbox. In fact, my daily self-care routine has evolved to become a source of energy and spiritual and mental fulfillment that I didn't think was possible before. After years of trial and error, I finally have a regimen that works for me.

After reading Hal Elrod's book, *The Miracle Morning*, I adopted the SAVERS strategy, a daily ritual of personalized self-care. The letters in the acronym stand for silence, affirmations, visualization, exercise, reading, and scribing (journaling). The structure imposed by having to get all these things done daily helps me prioritize my self-care, so that I can then go out and serve others. Many of us go after serving others first and end up having no energy to nourish our own soul. The strategy of SAVERS is to make sure to nourish your own body and mind first, so that you are ready and fit to help others. This new way of living, has helped me be a better medical professional, a better friend, parent and spouse. I have an abundance of energy after nourishing myself.

This life-changing practice has become the basis of a regular conversation I have with my patients, friends, and family because it's been so valuable to me. Whether I simply stretch out all my muscle groups, jog in place, or do sit-ups and crunches, it all counts as my exercise and movement for that day.

Small daily disciplines compound over time, just like investing in the stock market. The gains I have realized from small daily movement have been life changing. No one can see these actions building on each other, and sometimes they feel meaningless.

However, over time, these actions—if they are the right ones for you— build a life that is drastically different from what it was before. Give yourself time to see the difference. Doing the right actions can only help your cause, not hurt it.

# Chapter 4: Working Your Environment

*"If your environment is not to your liking, change it!"*

—*Napoleon Hill*

Is your house clean? Your physical house, your emotional house, your spiritual house?

Environment consists not only of our home, our physical surroundings, and our support system, but also the internal conversation we have with ourselves. Some aspects we can control, some we can't. We must build the most favorable environment possible in order to thrive despite our daily pain.

We have conversations in our minds from the time we wake up until the time we go to sleep. If you're not intentional about the conversation, it can go negative really quickly. One thought about what you can't do anymore or your frustration with a daily task that should be easy can send the mind into a spiral of negative thinking. And our minds are so powerful that left unchecked, these negative thoughts will grow into negative moods. Pretty soon, everything seems dismal and gloomy, even though nothing has actually changed. This also results in increased pain and fatigue—a vicious cycle that can be hard to pull yourself out of. But there's a lot you can do to stop this process.

Setting affirmation alerts on my phone for different periods throughout the day has been helpful for me. A positive reminder of what I'm grateful for or a quick reminder to focus on my current goal can snap me out of "stinking thinking" and replace it with a thought that serves me.

In the home environment, it can be easy to follow your old routines. Everything has a place, but sometimes the way you place things in your home doesn't serve the new you with chronic pain. Maybe it's a rug you constantly stumble over, or a cord in the middle of your walkway to the kitchen. Perhaps there is dust or spiderwebs in corners, causing your allergies to flare and make you feel worn down. Difficult, unpleasant conditions can cause suffering, as the following experience shows.

When I was diagnosed with fibromyalgia at age twenty-three, I had to move into a family apartment building with low rent so I could support myself. No one had lived there for several years, and I was aware a bathroom and kitchen sink would need to be installed. After all the construction, there was still a hole in the bathroom wall. Whenever anyone sat down on the toilet, they would have to turn sideways in order to not bump into the sink. The draft from the hole carried the damp smell of the unfinished portion of the basement.

At night, I could hear rats scurrying across the floor. After a couple of weeks of repeatedly cleaning off small black pellets from my soup cans, I realized it was rat poop and not just dirt all over them. I caught one large rat in a garbage bag and beat my broom against it until I was sure it was dead.

I cried myself to sleep that night, not sure what else I could do. How could I make this work? With the help of my new friend Toney, I hung blankets to keep the heat in the room I slept in. We attempted to plug the holes in the walls and set traps for the rats. It did make a difference. The small changes provided hope.

Most of us don't need to do a complete overhaul of our homes, but being creative about how to keep your body the most comfortable it can be in your space is vitally important. Creating a space to read, journal and meditate in your home is a small and inexpensive adjustment that can result in huge changes in your mood and energy. Chronic pain can be unpredictable. When and how much help you might need at any given point changes. It's important to nurture your support network so that it serves you. Be honest and vocal with family and friends about your boundaries and limitations when you aren't feeling well, but also let them know what you can manage to do and contribute yourself.

Many wives and moms with chronic pain and illness land in my exam room after burning themselves out trying to care for everyone in their lives. They push themselves to exhaustion to serve others. They feel guilty for taking a moment to themselves and feel obligated to sacrifice their needs for the well-being of spouses, children, and parents. They have the superwoman syndrome.

These super-givers end up crying in the shower, lying awake thinking all night, or being irritable and short with their families.

They can't pinpoint why they feel so bad. They don't realize they haven't nurtured their relationships. They haven't set boundaries or offered up what they prefer to help with.

But it needn't be this way for you. Family and friends who genuinely love you want to be supportive. Many find it difficult to know what to say or how to help. Seeing you in so much pain makes them feel helpless, as they're used to your strength and not your vulnerability.

But remember, it's your vulnerability that helps you build win-win relationships. Meet each person where they are emotionally and work from there. If a friend loves to cook, ask for simple, healthy meals. This creates the opportunity for them to give, and you don't have to worry about cooking. The friend who cooks may not be the ideal person with whom to discuss your frustration about your fatigue, however. Instead, share that with your aunt who loves to hear what's going on with you.

Despite your pain, you have more control than you realize. You get to decide how your internal conversation goes, how to configure your home to be a haven, and how to build mutually beneficial relationships with your support network based on honest and open communication.

Decide what all this looks like and get busy creating your ideal environment.

# Chapter 5: Difficult Relationships

*"We find comfort among those who agree with us—growth among those who don't."*

*—Frank A. Clark*

All of your roles—as a spouse and parent, an employee and colleague, a community leader or a church board member—every facet is affected by your physical capacity to perform well in that role.

Support is so important. When you have people around you who are understanding and compassionate, it can make the load of daily illness, fatigue, and depression more manageable, as you won't have to do everything alone.

Sometimes, for whatever reason, you may not have the appropriate support around you. Maybe you've overheard family members discussing your laziness and saying you exaggerate your pain. Maybe you're not invited anywhere because your friends feel as if you always have to cancel at the last minute.

Realizing what the raw feelings of others are toward you can be so emotionally scarring that your relationship with them is changed forever. This hurts, and there is no way around that. Not everyone will understand your new normal or believe your description of your pain.

The key is finding one person who gets it. This strategy has been a good start for me and many chronic pain warriors I have met. But you often feel a sense of guilt about the reliance you have on another human being when you have been diagnosed with a chronic pain disease.

Because many of these conditions have no observable disability, you don't look sick. Sometimes you try to mask your pain and fatigue to blend in and fit in with others. You can push your body beyond the limits to "prove" your commitment to giving your best on your good days. The consequence, though, is that after the push comes the crash—a flare-up of your symptoms that leaves you debilitated. A day of overexertion can cause weeks of recovery.

This push and crash cycle is exhausting on relationships. Though I have an incredible support network, the members of my household have the most exposure to my physical and emotional limits. We have to openly discuss boundaries and my need to protect my rest and sleep time. My one person has become my husband, Toney. I was diagnosed with fibromyalgia one year before we met. He knew what he was in for.

However, for some couples, the diagnosis comes after you've already built a life together. The transition to a new normal with a chronically ill spouse can be a challenge. Many patients can muster enough energy to perform for the outside world all day. But at home, people see the real you. The pain and fatigue after trying to keep your energy up all day is inevitable. So your spouse or children get whatever is left in your energy bank at the end of the day.

One way to manage this is to have guidelines to follow and commitments to each other. On rainy days, I tend to have an increase in pain and fatigue. My husband makes sure that he and my son are occupied quietly so I can always take a nap and let my body recover on those days. Since chronic pain flares are very unpredictable, making plans can be tricky. In order to support my husband, I try to do any task he has asked me to complete. I give myself a week's lead time, so that anytime during that week when I feel well, I can prioritize his request. We support each other, even though the way the support is carried out looks different from what you would see if chronic pain weren't a factor.

Get creative with your guidelines, boundaries, and commitments with your support team. Think of fun ways you can contribute. Try not to focus only on what you can do, not what you can't. This approach is more productive and gratifying in terms of your relationships than you could have ever imagined.

Let me know what your creative guidelines are on my Facebook page, @painfreepa or by email, contact@thepainfreepa.com

At twenty-six, Sara had a beautiful baby with curly brown hair and an infectious grin. She started coming to the eye clinic where I worked before becoming a physician assistant about one month after her baby was born. As a Type 1 diabetic, she had been used to having an invisible illness since she was a young girl. The insulin pump and multiple finger sticks to check her blood sugar were routine.

This new symptom of blurry vision and uncontrollable blood sugar was concerning, however, and she wanted to know what our retinal specialist could do to help improve her vision. My jaw dropped as she told me what he'd said. On the first meeting, the doctor had flatly stated, "I would have told you to never have a baby." Yet when she'd asked several doctors at the beginning of her pregnancy about possible complications from her diabetes, she had been told to keep her baby.

Hearing the retinal specialist's words was piercing to her. I watched her heart break as she sat in the chair and tears streamed down her face.

Several surgeries later, on both eyes, she could only see hand movements a few inches in front of her face. Finding her covered in feces after trying to change the baby's diaper, her family had to intervene. The loss of her sight presented challenges to her motherhood, but also to the management of her diabetes. Fortunately, a family member stepped up to take care of Sara and her young child. Our clinic helped with resources for low-vision patients.

When our health changes in a dramatic way, it can be difficult to navigate how family dynamics will change. Find one person who understands, and make sure you give wholeheartedly to building that alliance.

# Chapter 6: Ability Despite Disability

*"It is a waste of time to be angry about my disability. One has to get on with life and I haven't done badly. People won't have time for you if you are always angry or complaining."*

—*Stephen Hawking*

What do you do when you can't work? How do you support yourself? When I search for chronic pain forums and groups, I always find conversations about disability benefits.

At twenty-three, after being laid off from my customer service position at a telecom company, I was denied disability benefits. I needed a lawyer if I wanted to reapply. Seeing a young woman with no easily identifiable limitations, they practically laughed in my face and rolled their eyes at my pain.

I had to file for bankruptcy, as creditor calls were mounting. After my first rejection for supplemental food stamps, I received $141 per month with the appeal. I learned my Mercury Tracer was repossessed when I was going outside one morning to drop Toney off at work on my way to school. After that day, I took the bus to the community college for my ophthalmology technician courses.

The thing about feeling like a failure and being at your lowest point is that you can't fully appreciate all the opportunities around you. Though I was in school and on my way to having a better job, it was a daily mental battle to feel like a valuable member of the human race. There is no pride in needing assistance from anyone, let alone the government. Images of welfare queens and all the stereotypes I had grown up dodging landed squarely on my shoulders.

When you feel afflicted by something outside your control, like chronic pain and the accompanying depression, it can be hard to see your value and worth. I often had to ignore the whispers in my head: "Why bother? You won't be able to work with your pain," or "You'll never make it without government assistance—might as well quit school."

Have you ever heard those self-defeating whispers? Sure, most people have. The challenge is to remember that we come equipped to come to our own rescue. Our bodies recover from injury, remodel bones, and create and repair processes all day and night. Not only are our bodies incredibly made, but we've also proven over and over again that creativity and persistence can demolish any challenge. If you don't believe me, just look around. Humans were not made with wings, but we fly all over the world in airplanes. We are resourceful and always stretch the limits of imagination with invention and ingenuity.

Making the choice every day that I would work with patients and be compassionate with them, I would use all the customer service techniques I had learned and bring that skill to health care. Having been to eight doctors before receiving a diagnosis, I had so much experience as a patient that I wanted to help other patients as an advocate from the inside.

I couldn't afford to listen to disabling thoughts; there were people out there who needed me to become something for them. My husband and son were depending on me, but patients I hadn't yet met were depending on me too. Knowing this helped me put one foot in front of the other daily and keep going toward the goal.

Let's explore an example of how to reframe disability in your mind. I met Erica, a woman in her late thirties with chronic pain and fatigue. After her doctors had established a diagnosis of fibromyalgia and shared some helpful resources with her, she was doing very well. With exercise, meditation, and a nerve medication daily, she started to have a great life with more functional ability than she had experienced in years.

A year later, she told me she was having heart failure symptoms and her doctors couldn't figure out what was happening to her. Swollen legs, a heart rate of 130–140, and shortness of breath greeted her every morning when she was getting out of bed.

Her disabilities were mounting, but no one knew what would happen next. Erica could have become angry that doctors didn't have definitive answers or treatments. She could have become resigned to lie in bed and sink deeper into the depressing thoughts trying to invade her mind. She had kept meticulous records of her symptoms, heart rate changes, and weight. This could have consumed her and fed her anxiety about what was happening.

Instead, she reached out to me to brainstorm solutions. Her questions were based on a focus on what she could do, not what she couldn't. We talked about her passions, her fears, her missed opportunities from the life she'd wanted before she settled for the life she had. She decided to revisit a passion she had in the past, repurposing furniture out of flea market finds. She works for a few minutes and then rests when she needs to. She sells the pieces online and enjoys getting to spend more time with her son, who has special needs.

She turned her disability into a new life. A life beyond her chronic pain and illness. We are all different. Our new normal will be different, but the point is, every human has a contribution to make. No one is here as a placeholder. We all have a role to fill in this life, so turn your disability into an ability that serves you and the world around you.

Learning this principle has been transformative for so many. Take your time and really meditate on what you love to provide to the world or be in the world. Then get busy living the life you want despite the

limitations you saw before.

# Chapter 7: Ugly Stress

*"Stress is a form of suffering. Look at your body and see what stress does to the body and its functions—what it does to the heart, the circulation, the immune system, the digestive function, the liver."*

—*Eckhart Tolle*

The Valentine's Day Massacre took place in 2008 at my undergraduate school, Northern Illinois University (NIU). Our whole community was rocked when the gunman drove over three hundred miles to our school, opening fire in Wirtz Lecture Hall just after 3:00 p.m.

I left early that day, due to a stomachache. Pulling into my driveway at 3:00 p.m., I heard the helicopters buzzing above my apartment. When I turned on the news, my heart sank as the reporter on my television screen detailed the carnage. The perpetrator had opened fire with an assault weapon, killing five and wounding twenty-two students. Cell service was lost, so my anxious family members watched the news in horror, waiting to hear if I had been in the line of fire. Toney and Matthew rushed home to find me safe, and we hugged until my heartbeat stopped pounding in my chest.

The campus therapists were busy. Our community had been shaken and we all felt waves of grief without warning. Virginia Tech counselors and students had been through the same horrible experience the previous year. They came to support and offer guidance to this club we now belonged to as school shooting survivors.

I met Jay, a black psychologist with a large Afro, glasses, and curves like my mom's and aunts'. I instantly felt welcomed and at ease. My previous experiences with therapy always left me feeling misunderstood. She helped me see past the stigma of therapy, and past a mistrust of medical providers rooted in the mistreatment of generations of patients who looked like me.

Individual therapy and group therapy with my peers opened me up to a whole new world of release and communication I hadn't known before. My sleeping improved, I laughed more, and I was able to hug those victims of gunshot wounds limping through the hallways. I was learning to heal.

Stress and anxiety after trauma is understandable to most. We understand that combat veterans, domestic violence survivors, and gunshot victims have residual emotional pain long after the trauma itself has ended.

But what happens when we're going through small traumas and stressors every day?

The mind-body connection has become a mainstream term that draws attention to the fact that our thoughts can affect our physical health. Stress and anxiety actually take up most of the exam room conversations I have as a family medicine clinician.

Looking at my schedule daily, I make sure to have my nurses stock my exam rooms with two boxes of tissues. Our team knows that at least three patients per day will cry during their visit, regardless of why they came in for an appointment.

One such stressed patient was Cam. She had been experiencing fatigue and decreased energy for several months. Believing she had anemia or thyroid disease, she came to me asking for lab work. As I listened to her life routine and health history, more and more questions came up.

Cam was working fifty to sixty hours per week at her corporate job, managing her horse farm, and trying to coordinate calls with her daughter deployed overseas. Balancing these with all her other life chores was her daily mental obstacle course. Sleeping for about five hours per night, she never felt rested, but despite being tired she couldn't sleep any more than that.

Feeling exhausted and run down, she searched Google in an attempt to diagnose her symptoms. She was ready to hear that a deficiency in her minerals or hormones would explain how she was feeling. Before drawing any blood, we walked through her stressors and anxiety about her daughter. We came up with a plan and implemented stress reduction, counseling, and medication therapies that impacted her life immediately.

When we did get the lab results the following week, which were all normal, she was elated. Just discussing all the stressors and the effect they had on her sleep, her eating, her mood, and her attitude had made an impact. Cam went on to do presentations at her job and church regarding the importance of mental health and stress relief in maintaining a healthy body. She felt more energy and less pain daily as she did the emotional work to manage her stress.

Stress and mood changes are one of the least discussed topics when it comes to caring for chronic pain patients. The daily battle we wage in our minds is exhausting, so we need to explore how to handle stress effectively for ourselves. If you know stress is the main barrier to living a free life, it would be wise to take a deeper dive into the subject.

No one is immune to the effects of stress. Even after all my training and helping others overcome traumatic and stressful events, stress snuck up on me too. While living in California as a newly graduated physician assistant, I was excited to start seeing patients, but the road to California had been rough.

After graduating and taking my boards exam, my husband, six-year-old son, and I sat in the doctor's office awaiting the results of my husband's tonsil biopsy. We were sure the doctor would say they'd found a sunflower seed stuck inside, and that was what had caused his left tonsil to swell so much.

The surgeon asked if we wanted the nurses to tend to Matthew while we talked. Oblivious to his hint of the grave news to come, I declined. Matthew sat right beside me while the surgeon explained Toney's diagnosis: squamous cell carcinoma of the tonsil. My body was motionless with surprise as my husband looked at me, confused. He had no idea what those words meant. I whispered to him that it was cancer.

When the news came that I had passed my boards exam, I wanted to breathe a sigh of relief. I was thankful that I wouldn't have the embarrassment of telling my new boss that I couldn't start because I'd failed. Instead of experiencing relief, though, we scrambled to get Toney's surgery scheduled, as we were moving to California in three weeks.

Moving across the country to start a new position, I had to leave my recovering husband in North Carolina while I searched for a place to live in California. Starting a new career in a new state with a cancer survivor and a first grader who needed to be enrolled in school was daunting. I thought I was managing well, but a few months later I looked in the mirror and saw a thin and sickly body. I had lost thirty-eight pounds without trying.

Stress is sneaky. I thought I was being a boss and managing life well, but my body was absorbing all the negativity. Knowing the tools I used to help my patients did absolutely nothing to help me manage. Seeking out help from professionals was again a catalyst to getting back on track with eating and living well.

No one tool fits every person. If you're looking for help in exploring how to manage stress, check out my Facebook page for fellow chronic pain patients at @painfreepa

# Chapter 8: Breakdowns to Breakthroughs

*"People are more comfortable with a familiar discomfort than they are with an unfamiliar new possibility."*

*—Lisa Nichols*

Everyone has challenges. Without adversity and friction, it's difficult to grow as a human being. I have shared a few of my breakdowns in the preceding chapters, as well as some of my patients' struggles. Since you're reading this book, you have likely experienced some breakdowns as well. This is universal.

The difficulty for many with chronic pain, depression, and invisible illness is that sometimes the breakdowns are so frequent or so life changing that we can't see how to turn the breakdown into a breakthrough. Whether it's physical, emotional, or in our relationships, breakdowns can be tricky to navigate.

Kai, the patient with nine gunshot wounds, found his breakthrough after feeling listened to and understood. Cam found her breakthrough by embracing the connection between her mental health and her physical health. I've learned that sometimes I need another voice to help me get clear about what's happening. Usually a close friend or a therapist can help me think through how to pivot to a breakthrough.

So how do you change your "mess" into a message? What tools do you find serve you when trying to go from a negative situation to a positive mindset? Go ahead, take out a piece of paper or open up the notes app on your phone. Think through your breakdowns and how you rose out of them. How did you turn them into breakthroughs? If you're not sure, who will you get to help you think more clearly?

Many of my breakdowns have come surrounding money. Growing up, I always felt a sense of scarcity, of not enough to go around. There wasn't enough money for me to attend NIU, so I won scholarships and took out loans. Even with that, I was kicked out of school for a semester because I wasn't able to pay the balance. There wasn't enough money to live in a nice apartment, so I stayed with the rats and roaches, making do until I could do better.

Moving to North Carolina to attend Duke University for my master's as a physician assistant prompted my greatest money breakdown. My husband, Toney, agreed to quit his job to embark on this dream. We packed a U-Haul truck and drove twenty-four hours to Durham, North Carolina. I got the call three weeks before school was to start that my financial aid package was insufficient for me to attend.

Despite my 3.9 grade point average, scholarships, study experience abroad, and the honor societies on my resume, it was money that was the barrier. My credit was poor after filing bankruptcy. I wasn't able to get any graduate loans. I owed $16,429.32 and had three weeks to pay up.

After having my panicky moment and fearful thoughts of what to do next, I breathed. To come so close to my breakthrough, only to have it evaporate, seemed ludicrous. I centered myself and tried to think of a solution.

I sent out emails and made calls to all my counselors from NIU, my parents, and my extended family. Briefly, the thought crossed my mind to reach out to a couple, Lauren and Edward, I'd met at an NIU donor luncheon. At first I dismissed the thought, as they had only met me once, so they surely wouldn't remember me. Then gathering my courage, I hit send on the email to Lauren and Edward. As I prayed and cried, I was a little surprised to see a response a few hours later. Lauren sympathized and inquired about how much money I would need. After I told her the balance of $16,429.32, she let me know they would send me half. It was my job to work and get the rest.

Elated and grateful, I picked up the overnighted check and purchased my books, stethoscope, and first semester of training without knowing how I would continue.

My assigned advisor at Duke, the program director, called to discuss how I would proceed. She knew about the lack of financial aid and how big an obstacle I faced. With faith, I told her I planned to win the National Health Service Corps scholarship and she shouldn't worry about me.

Despite the confidence in my voice, I was on edge daily trying to learn all the information being poured into my brain while worrying about whether I'd be able to continue. Miraculously, on September 30th, six weeks after school started, I learned I was a recipient of the scholarship. In exchange for my promise to provide care in a medically underserved area, the scholarship would pay for all my school expenses and provide a monthly stipend for me to live off of. I would graduate from Duke with a zero balance.

The program director told me just before graduation how much my journey had increased her faith. When she'd first spoken to me on the phone, she was convinced I had a Pollyanna attitude about a very difficult situation. Now she understood that my faith had carried me to my destiny.

We all have stories we can point to that will increase our faith if we let them.

Remember I had you write down all your breakdowns and breakthroughs? You can see that in every situation you've been through, regardless of the outcome, you're now standing on the other side of it. You came through. The power of having survived a breakdown is found in making sure you learned from the situation and you've grown in strength from it.

The kindness shown to me was uncommon, but not really. Anyone who persistently seeks a solution to a breakdown finds a way to experience a breakthrough. The secret sauce is to keep going until you find the way. Just keep trying.

Share your breakdowns to breakthroughs with our community at the Painfree PA Facebook page, @painfreepa or the_pain_free_pa on Instagram.

# Chapter 9: Find Your Tribe

*"We are the sum of all the people we have ever met; you change the tribe and the tribe changes you."*

*—Dirk Wittenborn*

The word "tribe" has been gaining traction over the last few years. When someone identifies with your ideas, vision, and outlook on life, you're considered to be part of that person's tribe. We have heard all our lives that no one is an island, that we need each other to grow and develop into our best selves.

How do you know what tribe you belong to? The better question is, where do you feel at home?

Though I have many roles—wife, mother, woman, healer, and several others—my tribe that helps me feel at home consists of my family and a few close friends. Outside of that close circle, I am part of a mastermind group of women who brainstorm ideas and support each other's success. I also belong to the Motivating the Masses tribe of the transformational coach Lisa Nichols.

These tribes provide safe places for me to be uncensored and vulnerable, and to get all my emotional needs met. The people you lean on when you can't lean on your own limited knowledge about something are invaluable as you journey through life, especially if your journey is walking with chronic pain.

As mentioned earlier, when I was first diagnosed with fibromyalgia I went online to support groups. I went to physical therapy three times a week and took various medications for sleep, depression, and pain. At that time I was desperate to find people who had overcome the illness; I wanted a role model to follow. Unfortunately, I didn't find a mentor and I had to slowly build up helpful resources by trial and error.

Though I now have a great support team, I have also lost people I thought were forever friends, due to my physical and emotional limitations over the years. Have you ever lost friends due to having to cancel at the last minute, or not being able to keep commitments because you're physically unable? Sure, we all have. It hurts because you feel guilty, angry, and helpless to change this dynamic. But be reassured that you'll meet other members of your tribe.

Thankfully, the internet and access to information has advanced so much that connection to people hundreds, even thousands of miles away is possible and easier than ever before. Using the internet I have joined support groups not only for chronic pain, but also for budding authors and speakers, and groups for healers and medical professionals. For every role in my life, there are leaders and teachers online I can learn from. Many of them also become friends off-line too.

When *The Secret*, a documentary movie exploring the Law of Attraction and its role in creating specific outcomes, came out in 2006 and Lisa Nichols was one of the teachers from the movie featured on Oprah, it was the first time I saw someone like me beating adversity and achieving their dreams while serving others. As a black woman from inner city California and formerly on government assistance, she could probably identify with me, a Chicago girl on food stamps and turned down for disability who was trying to find a way to make it work.

When she talked about the Law of Attraction and thinking about what you want instead of what you don't want, it was completely foreign to me. Visualizing the life I wanted and taking action toward my goals weren't things I had seen anyone do consciously in real life, so I had some studying to do.

I devoured books about the Law of Attraction, the mind-body connection, and how to live the life you want. I listened to audiobooks in the car, watched YouTube videos about all the gurus in successful living, philosophy and psychology.

I raided the library for books on CD from Dale Carnegie, James Allen, Napoleon Hill, and so many others. These authors and thought leaders became mentors even though we never met.

Getting solution focused and reframing my thoughts toward positive outcomes resulted in my applying for and obtaining scholarships, getting invited to events with influential people, and having the opportunity to study abroad in China. In fact, it was in China that I learned the magnitude of having a global tribe and not being limited by what you see around you.

As a member of the Golden Key International Honor Society, I was invited on a medical delegation to China. We learned about their health care system and the practice of Traditional Chinese Medicine, and visited an autism center in a big city. It was amazing to watch cupping and acupuncture up close, but the most memorable aspect was meeting a rural farmer.

In the village of Xi'an, we were welcomed by a dragon dance in the rain. I was pulled in to participate and was surprised to splash across paved roads and to later enjoy the large feast they served us. We had heard the rural areas were much poorer than the urban centers. The government even allowed villagers to have more than one child (one is the law elsewhere in the country) so that farmers had enough help to work their land.

The farmer told us his story. He was the child of ostracized parents. Since they didn't agree with the Communist regime, they had a hard time finding employment. Their political beliefs ensured they could only be farmers; all other options for making a living were closed to them. As he spoke about the long days herding sheep on his family farm, he mentioned that he would paint to pass the time.

Through extensive practice, his paintings became masterpieces that were another source of income and acted as his ticket to travel the world. Despite his circumstances and the limitations he faced, he was able to provide paved roads and a hospital for his village through a hobby that turned to his calling.

The farmer always reminds me that no matter where you come from or what limitations you have, you can make a difference. Despite coming from the west side of Chicago and dodging bullets, rats, and roaches, I could make a difference. Despite having chronic pain, having to file for bankruptcy, and going through breakdown after breakdown, I could still contribute positively to the world and my community.

These are the people in my tribe: those who want to go after solutions and make the world better for all. I can identify with overcomers, and those who persevere despite evidence that it's an uphill climb.

Who is your tribe? Are you surrounded by them and feeling at home?

If not, what are you waiting for? Go find your tribe and be loved and supported as you deserve. People are waiting for you and your contribution.

# Chapter 10: Enlist the Medics

*"In successful relationships, perfection is the acceptance of imperfection."*

*—Wayne Gerard Trotman*

Medicine is an art, not a science. As I look at the landscape of medicine and our health care system in the United States, I can feel the skepticism in the minds of chronic pain patients. Many of us went to several doctors and medical professionals before receiving an accurate diagnosis. Some of us were told that the illness or illnesses we suffer from daily are "all in our minds." These experiences can set up an adversarial relationship with health care professionals.

Just as in any profession, there are excellent, adequate, and terrible medical providers. Just as we have to find our tribe, we have to find the providers who fit our style and offer a sense of security after the trauma of previous encounters. One of the reasons I chose to pursue medicine was that I wanted to help patients feel heard and understood. I am a patient who happens to also be a medical provider.

Practicing as a family medicine physician assistant has given me a unique view of patient care inside our current system. Though I have had the opportunity to help patients who feel disregarded or not believed by their health care providers, what was more surprising to me is the compassion I've developed for medical providers as well.

Working in Central Valley, California, in my first position as a physician assistant, I saw twenty-five to thirty-five patients in an eight-hour day. Sometimes there were two or even three patients scheduled in one fifteen-minute appointment slot. My patients were migrant farm workers and their families. They had limited access to care and often could not see a medical professional until it was unbearable to walk around with their conditions. Many were very ill. It was a routine occurrence to hear code blue over the intercom and rush to help someone who had passed out or needed immediate assistance.

Our normal appointment slots were fifteen minutes. In that time the nurse took the patient's vitals, copied their medication list, and recorded why they were being seen. In whatever time was left, I listened to their story, made an assessment, and came up with a plan. After seeing the other one or two patients sometimes scheduled in that same appointment slot, I had a moment to return to my desk, type notes in their charts, and send their medications. Of course this made the next patient wait a few more moments for me to enter the exam room and start the cycle again.

This workflow isn't uncommon in a family medicine practice. People are seen for viral colds, Pap smears, well-child checks, diabetes management, and everything else you can think of. So when a chronic pain patient is on the schedule, the medical provider may have to take a deep breath, as I did with Kai, before they pull their hair out from the frustration of knowing they don't have enough time to truly serve this patient.

One way to enlist the help of your medical provider in maximizing your care is to know how to do a doctor's visit. I'll provide some tips in the next section. I know,

I know—you're the patient and customer, and the appointment should be about the service you receive and being treated well. Remember, though, that just as your daily pain limits your best performance, doctors and health care professionals are suffering from burnout at alarming rates. The shortage of providers and our broken health care system are real problems that exist whether we accept it or not. Still, there are solutions available to you.

One excellent course of action is to maximize the time you do have with your provider and use all the resources available to you to live your healthiest life. To help you get the most from your visit with your healthcare provider, I have created The PainFree Visit document. To get a free copy to load onto your phone, please email me at contact@thepainfreepa.com

Oftentimes, a patient comes to a medical visit with a diagnosis and treatment plan they've googled at home. When you think about it, it's really not helpful to your cause. You're coming to your appointment to share symptoms or experiences you've had in the hopes of leaning on the expertise and experience of an evidence-based medical provider.

Though you're the expert on your body, your partner (the medical professional) has more data on patterns of outcomes in thousands of bodies. You have to work together as a team because neither of you have all the answers.

The presumed diagnosis you come in with will likely keep your medical provider thinking about that one possibility and not exploring all the other possibilities of what is happening with you. That puts you in a box concerning what will be treated versus an open field to be narrowed down by logic.

A more helpful approach to get the results you want is to have a plan and some flexibility. Go to your health care visits with a journal or notebook in which you've already written down the most important symptoms and a couple of closely related symptoms or questions. Be prepared to write down the answers you receive so you have a record of what recommendations were given. The next time you'll know if you followed the recommendations and if they worked.

Show your medical provider your list at the beginning of the visit. Sometimes they can address everything on your list by connecting all the dots, which lead to one diagnosis. Sometimes they can help you prioritize what is important during this visit and what can be addressed in a follow-up visit or a phone call.

This approach is a win-win, as the medical professional will actually feel that they have helped you and will want to continue to help with your progress. You both have objective information and don't have to guess what was communicated in each visit. We as humans can go off in tangents with talking, especially about all the aches, emotional changes, and relationship dynamics associated with chronic pain. Sometimes what you really need to talk about can be lost in the tangents. This approach helps you keep focused.

In addition, there are so many types health professionals now who can help patients maximize their experience. Companies and insurance plans have approved nutritionists, dieticians, social workers in employee assistance programs, and many more types of professionals. If your goal is to live the best life possible despite your chronic pain, utilize all the resources available to you and seek out new ones. This is your life to live—make the most of it.

# Getting The Most From This Book

Thank you for going on this journey with me. Action steps you can take right now to move closer to living a full life despite chronic pain and invisible illness are the following:

- Learn about your diagnosis, without becoming obsessed and depressed

- Develop a support network that serves you (and them).

- Write your self-care de-stress plan, and fill yourself up in order to give to others.

- Learn what dietary and exercise plans fit you.

- Find your tribe. You can join the PainFree Movement here @painfreepa

- Enjoy my FREE video series on 3 Action Steps to Thrive Despite Chronic Pain AND the Pain Free Doctors Visit guide to make the most out of your limited time in your medical appointments at www.thepainfreepa.com

**If you would like to work more closely with me to reframe Pain Free in your life with chronic pain and invisible illness sign up**

**for my online course to dive deeper into the
strategies in this book.**

contact@thepainfreepa.com



**If your organization needs an inspirational
keynote speaker, visit**

**to discuss how I can serve you.**

contact@thepainfreepa.com



The lessons you have learned in this
book can encourage and inspire you if you let
them. Read them over and over until they
become part of your DNA. As you become an
overcomer of pain and chronic disease, I
can't wait to hear your testimony. Join my

tribe on Facebook and Instagram. I look forward to hearing about your victories.

With love and light,

Michele Johnson MHS, PA-C

The PainFree PA